WORKBOOK

to accompany
STUDENT TUTOR CD-ROM

Kathleen A. Ireland

HUMAN ANATOMY
FOURTH EDITION

MARTINI / TIMMONS / TALLITSCH

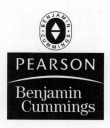

PEARSON

Benjamin
Cummings

San Francisco   Boston   New York
Capetown   Hong Kong   London   Madrid   Mexico City
Montreal   Munich   Paris   Singapore   Sydney   Tokyo   Toronto

Publisher: Daryl Fox
Executive Editor: Leslie Berriman
Project Editor: Kim Neumann
Editorial Assistant: Michael Roney
Managing Editor: Deborah Cogan
Cover Designer: Stacy Wong
Cover Art: Vincent Perez
Interior Designer: Kim Neumann
Manufacturing Buyer: Stacey Weinberger
Executive Marketing Manager: Lauren Harp

Screen captures appearing in labeling exercises courtesy of Visible Productions, LLC.
Illustrations courtesy of Dr. William C. Ober and Claire W. Garrison, R.N.

ISBN: 0-8053-5459-X

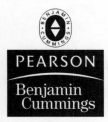

2 3 4 5 6 7 8 9 10 PBT 07 06 05 04
www.aw-bc.com

Preface

Given the quantity of new terms to learn and structures to locate, the science of anatomy can at times seem overwhelming. This workbook will assist you in your studies by bringing together the images and information in your *Human Anatomy*, **Fourth Edition** textbook and the images and animations on the Student Tutor CD-ROM, packaged with your new textbook. The possibilities for exploration of individual structures and entire systems offered by the combination of textbook, CD, and this workbook will allow you to build your three-dimensional understanding of the human body and develop an appreciation for its complexities and intricacies.

The exercises in this workbook are designed to reinforce scientific nomenclature and your functional understanding of anatomical concepts. They will also help you to link body systems to one another and to the entire organism. After the first chapter on the cell, the remaining chapters each focus on one of the body systems. All chapters begin with a list of **Learning Objectives** and a section titled **Core Concepts**, which presents a brief synopsis of the system. The variety of exercises and activities follow a sequence in each chapter that increases in complexity: **Labeling Exercise** to **Scavenger Hunt** to **Image Comparison**. The **Multiple Choice** questions at the end of the chapter check and support your understanding of key concepts.

This workbook will help you get the full benefits and value of the rich material on the Student Tutor CD-ROM.

Contents

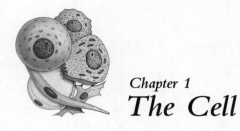

Chapter 1
The Cell

Learning Objectives

- Discuss the basic concepts of the cell theory.
- Explain the nature and importance of the cell membrane.
- Discuss how the structure of the membrane influences its function.
- Compare the structure and function of all the cellular organelles.
- Discuss the role of the nucleus as the cell's control center.
- Discuss how cells can be interconnected to maintain structural stability in body tissues.
- Describe the cell life cycle and how cells divide through the process of mitosis.

Core Concepts

All page references are to the fourth edition of Human Anatomy.

All living animals are composed of cells. The cell theory states that cells are: 1) the building blocks of all plants and animals; 2) produced from the division of preexisting cells; and 3) the smallest units that perform all vital functions (page 27). Cytology, the study of cells, provides us with a detailed look at the anatomy and physiology of individual cells.

Although there are many different types of cells in the human body, each selectively shares similar characteristics and structures (page 27). The typical cell includes a permeable outer membrane that separates the intracellular fluid from the extracellular, interstitial fluid. This membrane is composed of a phospholipid bilayer and includes peripheral and integral proteins functioning as channels (page 30). Substances entering or exiting the cell must pass across this membrane. Diffusion, osmosis, filtration, and facilitated diffusion are all passive transport mechanisms, moving substances across the cell membrane without expending energy (page 31). Active transport, endocytosis, and exocytosis require expenditure of ATP to move substances into or out of cells. Generally these processes move ions against their concentration gradient (page 32).

The cell's cytoplasm is found deep to the cell membrane (page 33). Cytoplasm is composed of cytosol, or intracellular fluid, and organelles. Organelles perform specific functions within the cell. The cytoskeleton, microvilli, centrioles, cilia, flagella, and ribosomes are all non-membranous organelles (page 34). These structures function in cellular support, division, and movement (either of fluids surrounding the cell or of the cell itself), or in the production of proteins. The membranous organelles are isolated from the cytosol by phospholipid membranes similar to the cell membrane (page 37). The nucleus, mitochondria, endoplasmic reticulum, Golgi apparatus, lysosomes, and peroxisomes fall into this category. The nucleus is covered by the nuclear envelope, which is studded with nuclear pores (page 38). Mitochondria are the site of ATP production (page 37). The endoplasmic reticulum, or ER, is a network of intracellular membranes involved in synthesis, storage, and transport of proteins and lipids (page 39). The Golgi apparatus packages materials for the lysosomes, peroxisomes and transport vesicles (page 40). Lysosomes are digestive vesicles, removing bacteria and debris from the cell (page 40). Peroxisomes break down organic molecules, neutralizing toxins (page 42).

The life cycle of most cells includes a period of growth alternating with a period of division (page 44). Growth is referred to as *interphase* and is divided into G1, S and G2 stages. Cell division, or mitosis, includes prophase, meta-phase, anaphase, and telophase (page 45). Mitosis is terminated with the completion of cytokinesis.

Labeling Exercise

Label the lettered structures, and then check your answers against the labeled image on the Student Tutor CD.

To locate the image, open your Student Tutor CD by launching the program and clicking **START**. Use the on-screen navigation menu and click through until you arrive at the **bold-face** item indicated.

Cell > Cell Flythrough

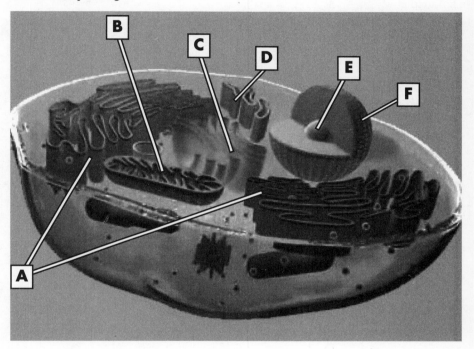

A. _____

B. _____

C. _____

D. _____

E. _____

F. _____

Scavenger Hunt

This activity offers a unique way for you to familiarize yourself with the location and functions of specific structures.

Open the Student Tutor CD by launching the program and clicking **START**. *Locate the structures displayed in* **boldface type** *below, and complete the questions that follow.*

1. Nucleus

What is the function of the nuclear structures represented as red dots on the surface of the nucleus?

2. Smooth endoplasmic reticulum

How does the function of this organelle compare with the function of the rough endoplasmic reticulum?

3. Mitochondrion inner membrane

How many compartments are in a mitochondrion, delineated by the outer and inner membranes?

4. Golgi apparatus

What is the relationship between the individual sacs of the Golgi apparatus?

Multiple Choice

This section gives you an opportunity to demonstrate your understanding of the material covered in this workbook and in the text. Circle the correct answer for each question.

1. Which of the following is NOT part of the cell theory?

    a. All cells come from pre-existing cells.

    b. Cells perform all vital functions.

    c. All cells have nuclei.

    d. Cells are the building blocks of both plants and animals.

2. The organelle involved in cholesterol synthesis is the

    a. rough endoplasmic reticulum.

    b. Golgi apparatus.

    c. lysosome.

    d. smooth endoplasmic reticulum.

3. The cell membrane is

    a. selectively permeable.

    b. composed of phospholipids arranged in a single layer.

    c. incomplete, allowing all substances to enter or exit the cell via pores.

    d. only composed of channel proteins and a glycocalyx.

4. The inner membrane of the mitochondrion is the site of

    a. cholesterol synthesis.

    b. protein synthesis.

    c. ATP synthesis.

    d. ribosome formation.

5. The nucleus houses

    a. DNA.

    b. RNA.

    c. the nucleolus.

    d. all of the above.

6. The organelle responsible for the digestion of cellular debris is the

   a. lysosome.
   b. nucleus.
   c. centriole.
   d. peroxisome.

7. Active transport mechanisms include:

   a. ion exchange pumps and facilitated diffusion.
   b. facilitated diffusion and filtration.
   c. osmosis and filtration.
   d. ion exchange pumps and receptor-mediated endocytosis.

8. On the CD, the organelle depicted as a ribbon-like structure with associated red dots within the cytoplasm of the cell is the

   a. smooth endoplasmic reticulum.
   b. rough endoplasmic reticulum.
   c. Golgi apparatus.
   d. centriole.

9. Interphase is divided into _____ stage(s).

   a. 1
   b. 2
   c. 3
   d. 4

10. The stage of cell division in which the daughter chromosomes are separated from one another is

   a. metaphase.
   b. telophase.
   c. prophase.
   d. anaphase.

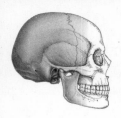

Chapter 2
The Skeletal System

Learning Objectives

- Describe the functions of the skeletal system.
- Compare the structures and functions of compact and spongy bone.
- Discuss the steps involved in the processes of bone development and bone growth.
- Classify bones according to their shape and give examples for each type.
- Identify the bones of the axial skeleton and describe their functions.
- Identify the bones, sutures, and bone markings of the skull.
- Describe the nasal complex and the functions of the individual elements.
- Distinguish differences among the skulls of infants, children, and adults.
- Describe the general structure and spinal curves of the vertebral column.
- Describe the features and landmarks of a representative rib.
- Identify the bones and surface features of the pectoral girdle and upper limb.
- Identify the bones and surface features of the pelvic girdle and lower limb.
- Distinguish among the different types of joints.
- Link anatomical design to joint functions and describe accessory structures.
- Describe the dynamic movements of the skeleton.
- Describe the six types of synovial joints based on their movement.

Core Concepts

All page references are to the fourth edition of Human Anatomy.

The skeletal system is composed of the bones of the skeleton, as well as the cartilages, ligaments, and connective tissues that stabilize them. Functions of the skeletal system include: support; storage of minerals and lipids; blood cell production; protection; and leverage (page 113).

Bone is composed of osseous tissue. The vast majority of osseous tissue is comprised of calcium ions embedded in a hard matrix of hydroxyapatite. Collagen fibers within the matrix provide flexible strength (page 113). Cells make up less than 2% of the total volume of bone. There are four types of cells found in bone: osteocytes, osteoblasts, osteoprogenitor cells, and osteoclasts (Page 113). Histologically bone can be arranged in osteons (compact bone) or in trabeculae (spongy or cancellous bone) (page 114). The regions of a long bone include the epiphysis, the diaphysis, and the marrow cavity. Bone is covered by periosteum, and the marrow cavity is lined with endosteum (page 117).

Bone can be formed in one of two ways: by intramembranous ossification (page 118) or by endochondral ossification (page 120). Normal bone growth is regulated by nutritional and hormonal factors.

Bone shape can be classified as long, short, flat, irregular, sesamoid, or sutural (page 126). Each bone of the body has a distinctive shape and characteristic features. These features are created where tendons and ligaments attach, where adjacent bones articulate, and where blood vessels and nerves penetrate or lie along the bone surface (page 128).

The skeleton is composed of two divisions: the axial and appendicular. The axial skeleton is made up of 80 bones and includes the skull and associated bones, the thoracic cage, and the vertebral column (page 134). The appendicular skeleton is made up of 126 bones, and consists of the pectoral girdle and upper limbs, and the pelvic girdle and lower limbs (page 181).

Articulations, or joints, connect the bones of the skeletal system. Joints can be classified based on structure or degree of motion. Structurally, joints can be classified as hinge joints, gliding joints, pivot joints, saddle joints, ellipsoidal joints, or ball-in-socket joints (page 221). Pages 222–238 in the text provide detailed descriptions of representative joints from each of these categories.

Individual variations in the skeletal system can be caused by gender differences, dietary differences, differences in average body size, muscle mass, and muscular strength (page 209).

Labeling Exercise #1

Label the lettered structures, and then check your answers against the labeled image on the Student Tutor CD.

To locate the images in the exercises that follow, open your Student Tutor CD by launching the program and clicking **START**. Use the on-screen navigation menu and click through until you arrive at the **boldface** item indicated.

Skeletal System > Axial > Skull Base (view from top)

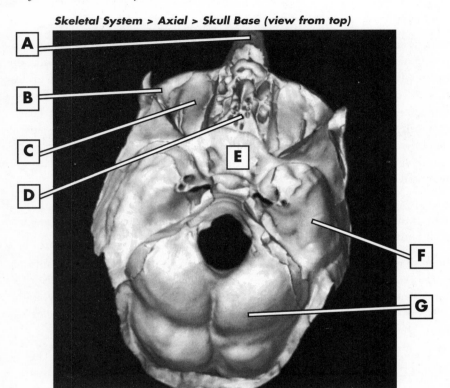

A. _____

B. _____

C. _____

D. _____

E. _____

F. _____

G. _____

Labeling Exercise #2

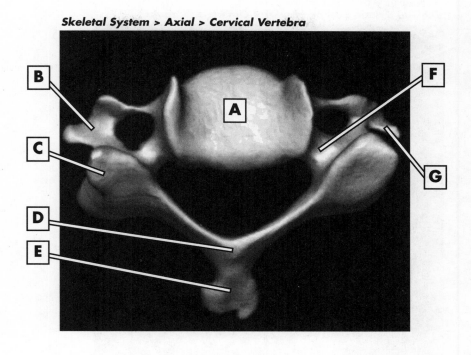

Skeletal System > Axial > Cervical Vertebra

A. _____

B. _____

C. _____

D. _____

E. _____

F. _____

G. _____

Labeling Exercise #3

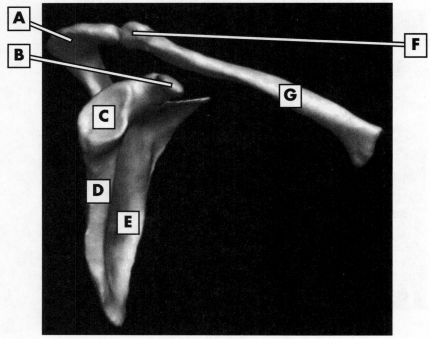

A. _____

B. _____

C. _____

D. _____

E. _____

F. _____

G. _____

Labeling Exercise #4

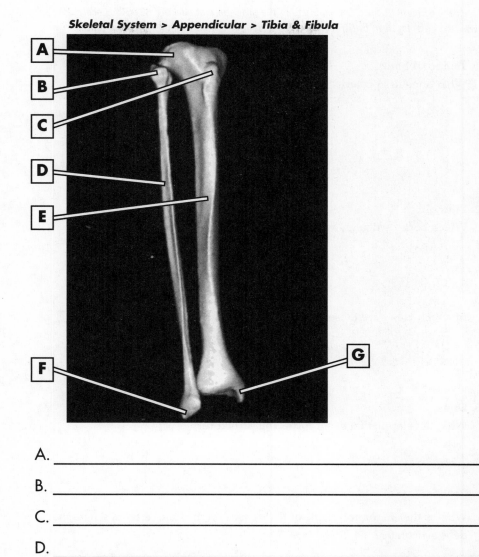

Skeletal System > Appendicular > Tibia & Fibula

A. _____

B. _____

C. _____

D. _____

E. _____

F. _____

G. _____

Scavenger Hunt

This activity offers a unique way for you to familiarize yourself with the location and functions of specific structures.

Open the Student Tutor CD by launching the program and clicking **START**. *Locate the structures displayed in* **boldface type** *below, and complete the questions that follow.*

1. Temporal bone

What bone lies posterior to the temporal bone, near the spinal cord?

2. Ethmoid

Which bones articulate with the ethmoid?

In which views are these bones most easily seen?

3. Dens

What developmental event forms this structure?

What is the anatomical name of the surface on the first vertebra where the dens articulates?

4. Ala

Which bones does the ala come into contact with at the lateral auricular surfaces?

5. Medial Epicondyle of the Humerus

What structure lies over the medial epicondyle?

How does this structure differ from the condyle immediately lateral to it?

6. Acetabulum

Which hip bones compose the acetabulum?

What is unique about this joint?

7. Talus

Which bones articulate with the talus?

8. Vomer

Which bones articulate with the vomer?

What injury would you have to sustain in order to break the vomer?

9. Trochlear notch

What structure lies distal to the trochlear notch?

What bone lies proximal to the trochlear notch?

10. Patellar surface

What bone lies superficial to the patellar surface?

Image Comparison

Looking at anatomical structures from many perspectives enables you to learn their general organization and specific structures. By comparing your textbook's illustrations with the 3-dimensional art on the Student Tutor CD, you will sharpen your ability to identify these structures.

Open the Student Tutor CD by launching the program and clicking START. Look at the corresponding images from the CD and textbook listed before each set of questions, then answer the questions.

1. CD: Skeletal System > Axial > Exploded Skull
   Textbook: Figure 6.9

   a. What suture are you looking through to see the sphenoid?

   b. Which bones articulate with the sphenoid?

   c. What does the exploded skull view allow you to see?

2. CD: Skeletal System > Axial > Skull
   Textbook: Figure 6.15

   a. What cranial bone lies posterior to the orbital complex?

b. What structure are you looking through to see this bone on the CD?

c. Which bones make up the orbital complex?

3. CD: Skeletal System > Axial > Rib Cage
   Textbook: Figure 6.27

   a. Describe the attachment of the ribs to the thoracic vertebrae. Are the ribs articulating at the superior or inferior surface of the vertebra?

   b. Using the CD, describe the relationship between the ribs, vertebra, and sternum.

4. CD: Skeletal System > Appendicular > Clavicle and Scapula
   Textbook: Figure 7.5c

   a. How does the clavicle relate to the coracoid process and the acromion of
   the scapula? Which image source provides this detail best?

5. CD: Skeletal System > Appendicular > Humerus
   Textbook: Figure 7.6

   a. How does the intertubercular sulcus, or groove, relate to the anatomical
   neck of the humerus?

   b. Is the shaft of the humerus straight or bowed? Which angle best
   demonstrates this on the CD?

Multiple Choice

This section gives you an opportunity to demonstrate your understanding of the material covered in this workbook and in the text. Circle the correct answer for each question.

1. **The portion of bone matrix that provides the flexible framework of the bone is the**

    a. hydroxyapatite.
    b. collagen fibers.
    c. osteocytes.
    d. osseous tissue.

2. **The opposing ends of long bones in synovial joints are covered with**

    a. periosteum.
    b. synovial lining.
    c. articular cartilage.
    d. epiphyses.

3. **The functions of the periosteum include all of the following EXCEPT**

    a. creating red marrow.
    b. isolating and protecting bone.
    c. providing a place of attachment for nerves.
    d. assisting in growth and repair.

4. **Dermal bones include the**

    a. frontal bone.
    b. mandible.
    c. femur.
    d. both A and B.

5. **Endochondral ossification begins with**

    a. a nutrient artery penetrating an area and creating bone.
    b. a hyaline cartilage model of the bone.
    c. the formation of epiphyses and diaphyses.
    d. calcium deposition in loose connective tissue.

6. The carpal bone that articulates with metacarpal I is the

    a. trapezoid bone.

    b. hamate bone.

    c. trapezium.

    d. triquetrum.

7. The three bones that fuse to form one os coxae are the

    a. acetabulum, ilium, and pubis.

    b. ilium, ischium, and pubis.

    c. ischium, acetabulum, and sacrum.

    d. sacrum, acetabulum, and symphysis.

8. The portion of the femur in direct contact with the os coxae is the

    a. acetabulum.

    b. greater trochanter.

    c. head.

    d. lesser trochanter.

9. The largest of the tarsal bones is the

    a. talus.

    b. navicular bone.

    c. tibia.

    d. calcaneous.

10. The joint found between the atlas and axis is best described as

    a. a pivot joint.

    b. a gliding joint.

    c. an ellipsoid joint.

    d. none of the above.

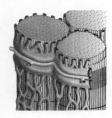

Chapter 3
The Muscular System

Learning Objectives

- Describe the functions of skeletal muscle.
- Discuss the organization of skeletal muscle.
- Describe the cellular arrangement of skeletal muscle fibers.
- Discuss the events of the neuromuscular junction during action potential transmission.
- Summarize the process of muscular contraction.
- Describe a motor unit and control of muscle fibers.
- Describe the different classes of levers.
- Explain how muscles interact to produce or oppose movement.
- Identify and locate the principle axial muscles of the body.
- Describe the origins and insertions of the axial muscles.
- Describe the innervations and actions of axial muscles.
- Describe the functions of the appendicular musculature.
- Identify and locate the principle appendicular muscles of the body.
- Define the origins and insertions of appendicular muscles.
- Describe the innervations and actions of appendicular muscles.
- Compare the major muscle groups of the upper and lower limbs.

Core Concepts

All page references are to the fourth edition of Human Anatomy.

The Muscular System is composed of skeletal muscle. It provides five functions for the body: (1) produces skeletal movement; (2) maintains posture and body position; (3) supports soft tissues; (4) regulates entering and exiting of material; and (5) maintains body temperature. The four basic properties of skeletal muscle are excitability, contractility, extensibility, and elasticity (page 245).

Muscles are composed of three concentric layers of connective tissue: the epimysium, perimysium, and endomysium (page 245). Skeletal muscle fibers are multinucleate and include T-tubules on their sarcolemma, which conduct electrical impulses. Myofibers contain hundreds of myofibrils with each myofibril surrounded by the sarcoplasmic reticulum. The ends of this SR are swollen into terminal cisternae, important in contraction. The myofilaments actin and myosin are arranged within myofibers in regular patterns called sarcomeres, which make up the contracting unit of the muscle (page 247).

Muscle contraction occurs via the sliding filament theory (page 251) and is controlled by motor neurons at the neuromuscular junction (page 253). The bones and muscles of the body work as levers. There are first class, second class, and third class levers, classified by the relative positions of the fulcrum, resistance, and force (page 259).

Muscles of the body can be divided into axial or appendicular muscles (page 267). The muscles of the head and neck can be grouped into muscles of facial expression (page 269), extra-occular muscles (page 271), muscles of mastication (page 273), tongue (page 274), pharynx (page 275), and anterior muscles of the neck (page 276). The muscles of the vertebral column adjust the position of the vertebral column, head, neck, and ribs (page 278). The oblique and rectus muscles compress underlying structures between the vertebral column and the ventral midline and assist in moving the trunk (page 281). The muscles of the pelvic floor form the urogenital triangle and anal triangle (page 284).

The appendicular muscles are grouped into muscles of the pectoral girdle and upper limbs, and muscles of the pelvic girdle and lower limbs. Pectoral girdle and upper limb muscles are further subdivided into muscles that position the pectoral girdle (page 292), muscles that move the arm (page 295), muscles that move the forearm and hand (page 297), and muscles that move the hand and fingers (page 299). The muscles of the pelvic girdle and lower limb are subdivided into muscles that move the thigh (page 305), muscles that move the leg (page 309), and muscles that move the foot and toes (page 313).

Labeling Exercise #1

Label the lettered structures, and then check your answers against the labeled image on the Student Tutor CD.

To locate the images in the exercises that follow, open your Student Tutor CD by launching the program and clicking **START**. Use the on-screen navigation menu and click through until you arrive at the **boldface** item indicated.

Muscular System > Axial > Head & Face

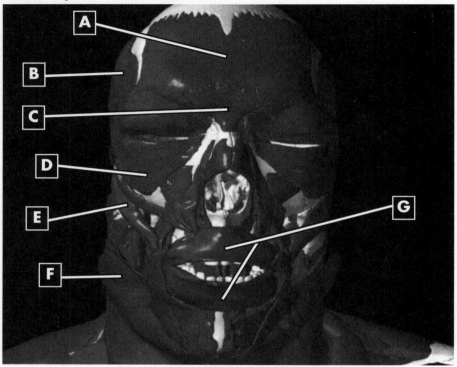

A. _____

B. _____

C. _____

D. _____

E. _____

F. _____

G. _____

Labeling Exercise #2

Muscular System > Axial > Thorax & Abdomen (posterior view)

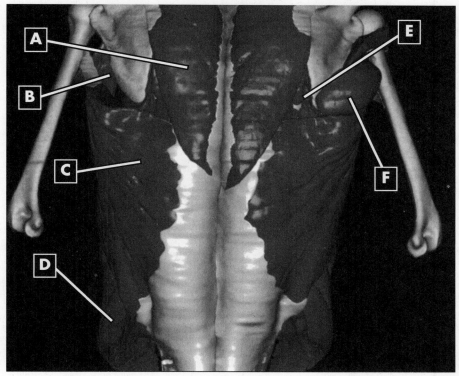

A. _____

B. _____

C. _____

D. _____

E. _____

F. _____

Labeling Exercise #3

Muscular System > Appendicular > Shoulder & Upper Arm

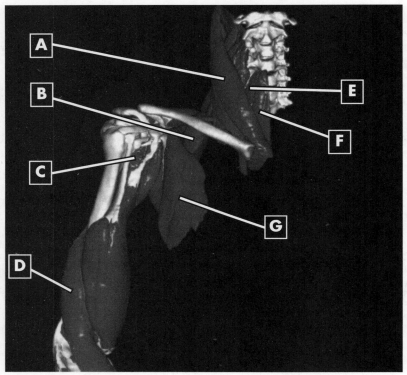

A. _____

B. _____

C. _____

D. _____

E. _____

F. _____

G. _____

Labeling Exercise #4

Muscular System > Appendicular > Thigh

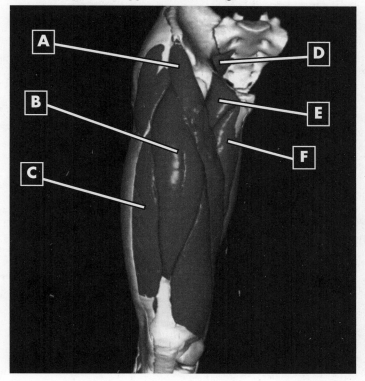

A. _____

B. _____

C. _____

D. _____

E. _____

F. _____

Scavenger Hunt

This activity offers a unique way for you to familiarize yourself with the location and functions of specific structures.

Open the Student Tutor CD by launching the program and clicking **START**. *Locate the structures displayed in* **boldface type** *below, and complete the questions that follow.*

1. Vastus intermedius muscle

What structure lies immediately superficial to the vastus intermedius muscle?

2. Extensor hallucis longus muscle

What muscle lies medial to the extensor hallucis longus muscle?

3. Middle scalene muscle

What muscle lies obliquely across the middle scalene muscle?

4. Biceps brachii tendon

What muscle lies superficial to the biceps brachii tendon?

5. Pronator teres muscle

Which muscles lie deep to the pronator teres muscle?

6. Flexor pollicus longus muscle

What structure does the flexor pollicus longus muscle lead to, and lie against?

7. Coracobrachialis muscle

To what structures does the coracobrachialis muscle attach?

8. Depressor anguli oris muscle

Which muscles lie medial to the depressor anguli oris muscle?

9. Occipitalis muscle

What bone is deep to the occipitalis muscle?

10. Quadratus lumborum muscle

What structure lies medial to the quadratus lumborum muscle?

Image Comparison

Looking at anatomical structures from many perspectives enables you to learn their general organization and specific structures. By comparing your textbook's illustrations with the 3-dimensional art on the Student Tutor CD, you will sharpen your ability to identify these structures.

Open the Student Tutor CD by launching the program and clicking **START**. *Look at the corresponding images from the CD and textbook listed before each set of questions, then answer the questions.*

1. CD: Muscular System > Axial > Head & Neck
   Textbook: Figure 10.3

   a. Where is the the procerus muscle located? Describe its appearance in the two images.

   b. Describe the relationship between the masseter muscle, the risorius muscle and the platysma. Which image provides a more complete understanding of the relationships between these muscles?

2. CD: Muscular System > Axial > Thorax & Abdomen
   Textbook: Figure 10.13

   a. What are the three layers of muscle that protect and cover the abdominal area?

   b. How are these muscles related to one another?

   c. What muscle can be identified immediately deep to the internal oblique muscles, visible where the rectus sheath meets this muscle?

3. CD: Muscular System > Appendicular > Arm
   Textbook: Figure 11.6

   a. Look closely at these two images. Compare them and list the structures that are identical.

b. Now find the differences between the two depictions and list them below.

4. CD: Muscular System > Appendicular > Thigh (second screen, view of deep muscles)
   Textbook: Figure 11.10

   a. Describe the locations of the piriformis muscle and the quadratus femoris muscle.

   b. What are the main functions of these two muscles?

   c. What muscles lie along the length of the femur? Why are these not visible in Figure 11.10?

Multiple Choice

This section gives you an opportunity to demonstrate your understanding of the material covered in this workbook and in the text. Circle the correct answer for each question.

1. A fascicle is a

    a. muscle.

    b. bundle of muscle fibers enclosed by a connective tissue sheath.

    c. bundle of myofibrils enclosed by a connective tissue sheath.

    d. group of myofilaments.

2. The sites where the motor nerve impulse is transmitted to the skeletal muscle cell is the

    a. sarcomere.

    b. motor unit.

    c. neuromuscular junction.

    d. T-tubules.

3. Characteristics of thick filaments include

    a. myosin proteins.

    b. tropomyosin and troponin.

    c. actin active sites.

    d. calcium binding proteins.

4. The function of the corrugator supercilii muscles is to

    a. squint the eyes.

    b. raise the eyebrows.

    c. smile.

    d. pucker the lips.

5. The quadriceps muscle group includes all of the following EXCEPT

    a. vastus lateralis muscle.

    b. biceps femoris muscle.

    c. rectus femoris muscle.

    d. vastus intermedius muscle.

6. **The rhomboid major muscle moves the**

   a. scapula.
   b. clavicle.
   c. humerus.
   d. ulna.

7. **The functions of the latissimus dorsi muscle include**

   a. extension at the shoulder.
   b. medial rotation at the shoulder.
   c. abduction at the shoulder.
   d. A and B are correct.

8. **The term "pollicis" refers to the**

   a. great toe.
   b. small toe.
   c. thumb.
   d. small finger.

9. **The piriformis muscle originates on the _____ and inserts on the _____ .**

   a. femur; sacrum
   b. sacrum; femur
   c. ischium; femur
   d. pubis; sacrum

10. **The muscles of the hamstrings include all of the following EXCEPT**

   a. adductor magnus muscle.
   b. semimembranosus muscle.
   c. biceps femoris muscle.
   d. semitendinosus muscle.

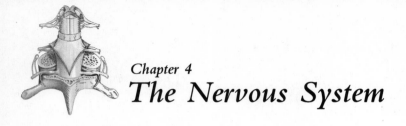

Chapter 4
The Nervous System

Learning Objectives

- Discuss the structure and functions of the spinal cord.
- Locate the spinal meninges, describe their structure, and list their functions.
- Identify the regional groups of spinal nerves.
- Identify the four main spinal nerve plexuses.
- Describe the structures and steps involved in a neural reflex.
- Name the major regions of the brain and describe their functions.
- Describe the structural and functional characteristics of the choroid plexus.
- Identify the anatomical structures and functions of the cerebrum.
- Identify the structuresand functions of the thalamus and hypothalamus.
- Identify the major features and functions of the mesencephalon.
- Identify the components and functions of the cerebellum.
- Identify the anatomical structures and functions of the medulla oblongata.
- Identify and describe the twelve cranial nerves.
- Identify the centers in the brain that determine somatic motor output.
- Describe the regions of the brain involved in memory storage and recall.
- Explain the structure and function of the reticular activating system.
- Compare the autonomic nervous system (ANS) with the rest of the nervous system.
- Identify the principal structures and the two functional divisions of the ANS.
- Describe the anatomy of the sympathetic division.
- Describe the anatomy of the parasympathetic division.
- Identify and give the functions of the receptors for the general senses.
- Discuss the receptors and neural pathways involved in the sense of taste.
- Describe the mechanism by which we maintain equilibrium.
- Describe pathways taken by auditory/equilibrium information.
- Identify the layers of the eye and the structures of the visual pathway.

Core Concepts

All page references are to the fourth edition of Human Anatomy.

The nervous system has two anatomical divisions: the central nervous system (CNS) and the peripheral nervous system. The central nervous system includes the spinal cord and brain. It is responsible for integrating, processing, and coordinating sensory data and motor commands. The peripheral nervous system includes all neural tissue outside the CNS. It provides sensory information to the CNS and carries motor commands from the CNS (page 335).

The spinal cord is located in the vertebral canal. It has a layer of white matter covering the central gray matter. In gross anatomy, the cord has two enlargements: the cervical enlargement and the lumbosacral enlargement (pages 356–357). It ends at L_1 at the conus medullaris. Extending beyond that is the cauda equina and the filum terminale (pages 356–357). Three layers of meninges cover the spinal cord. From exterior to interior they are the dura mater, the arachnoid, and the pia mater (page 356). Spinal nerves extend from the spinal cord at regular intervals (page 362). These nerves are mixed nerves, carrying both sensory and motor information (page 364). The cervical plexus integrates information from the cervical region (page 364). The brachial plexus integrates information from the upper limbs, and the lumbosacral plexus integrates information from the lower limbs (page 367). Reflexes, both innate and acquired, are immediate involuntary motor responses to specific stimuli (page 373). They involve the spinal cord, and usually include a receptor, a sensory neuron, an interneuron within the gray matter of the cord, a motor neuron, and an effector organ (page 373).

The brain is housed in the cranium. It is composed of six major regions: the cerebrum, the diencephalon, the mesencephalon, the pons, the cerebellum, and the medulla oblongata (page 382). The general functions of these regions are described on pages 391–409.

There are 12 cranial nerves extending from the underside of the brain. They are the olfactory, optic, oculomotor, trochlear, trigeminal, abducens, facial, vestibulocochlear, glossopharyngeal, vagus, accessory, and hypoglossal nerves (pages 410–418).

The senses are divided into the general senses and the special senses. General senses include exteroceptors, interoceptors, and proprioceptors (page 468). The special senses include olfaction, gustation, vision, hearing, and equilibrium. The special senses are described in detail on pages 472–497.

Labeling Exercise #1

Label the lettered structures, and then check your answers against the labeled image on the Student Tutor CD.

To locate the images in the exercises that follow, open your Student Tutor CD by launching the program and clicking **START**. Use the on-screen navigation menu and click through until you arrive at the **boldface** item indicated.

Nervous System > Brain (right-side view, cross-section)

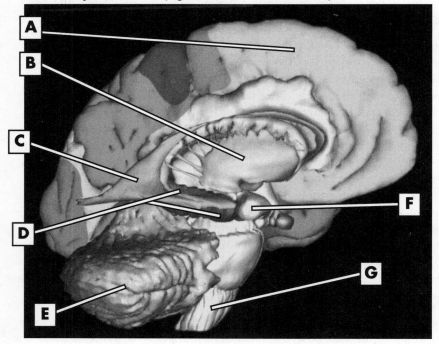

A. _____

B. _____

C. _____

D. _____

E. _____

F. _____

G. _____

Labeling Exercise #2

Nervous System > Spinal Cord (second level deep)

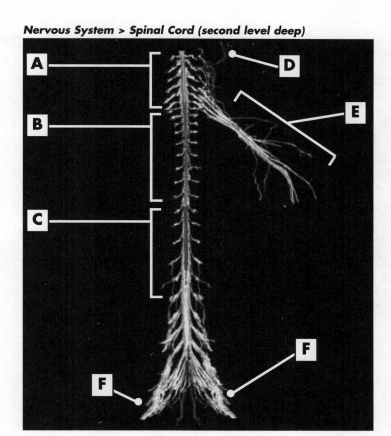

A. _____

B. _____

C. _____

D. _____

E. _____

F. _____

Labeling Exercise #3

Nervous System > Eye: Coronal Interior (second level deep, cross-section)

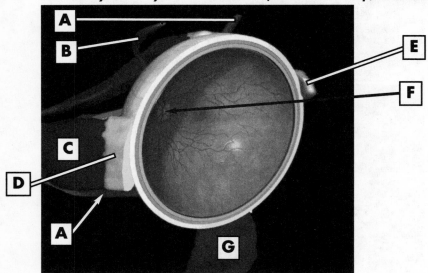

A. _____

B. _____

C. _____

D. _____

E. _____

F. _____

G. _____

Scavenger Hunt

This activity offers a unique way for you to familiarize yourself with the location and functions of specific structures.

*Open the Student Tutor CD by launching the program and clicking **START**. Locate the structures displayed in **boldface type** below, and complete the questions that follow.*

1. Ventricles of the brain

What fluid originates at the ventricles of the brain and what is its function?

What structures are inferior and medial to the lateral ventricles?

2. Wernicke's language area

Which areas lie between Wernicke's language area and Broca's speech area?

3. Cauda equina

The cauda equina extends between what levels of the vertebral column?

Which medical procedures are possible in this area of the spinal cord?

4. Lumbosacral plexus

What nerves originate in the lumbosacral plexus?

5. Lens of the eye

What is the anatomical name of the structure indicated on the CD as holding the lens of the eye in place?

6. Hippocampus

What structures lie adjacent to the hippocampus?

7. Ophthalmic nerve

Describe the anatomical relationship between the ophthalmic nerve and the optic nerve.

8. Tibial nerve

The tibial nerve branches from which larger plexus?

What nerves lie medial to the tibial nerve?

Image Comparison

Looking at anatomical structures from many perspectives enables you to learn their general organization and specific structures. By comparing your textbook's illustrations with the 3-dimensional art on the Student Tutor CD, you will sharpen your ability to identify these structures.

*Open the Student Tutor CD by launching the program and clicking **START**. Look at the corresponding images from the CD and textbook listed before each set of questions, then answer the questions.*

1. **CD: Nervous System > Spinal Cord**

   Textbook: Figure 14.1

   a. Describe the location and appearance of the conus medullaris. Does the conus medullaris appear similar on both images?

2. **CD: Nervous System > Brain (third level deep)**

   Textbook: Figure 15.9

   a. What is the anatomical location of the somatic sensory association area on the brain?

b. Do both images give the same information, or is one more complete than the other?

3. CD: Nervous System > Ear (third level deep)
Textbook: Figure 18.9

a. Trace the pathways of the facial nerve as viewed through the ear.

b. Which image is more helpful in this task? Explain why.

Multiple Choice

This section gives you an opportunity to demonstrate your understanding of the material covered in this workbook and in the text. Circle the correct answer for each question.

1. The white matter of the central nervous system is arranged in

    a. tracts and columns.
    b. plexuses.
    c. ganglia.
    d. bundles of axons.

2. The expanded area of the cord that supplies nerves to the pelvic girdle and lower limbs is the

    a. conus medullaris.
    b. filum terminale.
    c. lumbar enlargement.
    d. cervical enlargement.

3. The major nerves of the brachial plexus include all of the following EXCEPT

    a. musculocutaneous nerve.
    b. median nerve.
    c. radial nerve.
    d. common fibular nerve.

4. The tough outer meninge that protects both the spinal cord and the brain is the

    a. dura mater.
    b. arachnoid.
    c. pia mater.
    d. epidural space.

5. The correct sequence of cells through which light passes is

    a. rods and cones > ganglion cells > bipolar cells.
    b. rods and cones > bipolar cells > ganglion cells.
    c. ganglion cells > bipolar cells > rods and cones.
    d. bipolar cells > rods and cones > ganglion cells.

6. The area of greatest visual acuity is the

a. fovea centralis.

b. optic disc.

c. central retinal blood vessels.

d. canal of Schlemm.

7. Olfactory receptors respond to

a. dissolved compounds in the mouth that aerate up through the nasopharynx.

b. dissolved compounds that are carried into the nose with a breath.

c. solid compounds that pass the nasal epithelium.

d. A and B are correct.

8. The cardiovascular center and the respiratory rhythmicity centers are located in the

a. medulla oblongata.

b. pons.

c. cerebellum.

d. cerebrum.

9. The separation between the two hemispheres of the cerebrum is the

a. squamous suture.

b. fornix.

c. longitudinal fissure.

d. frontal lobe.

10. The functions of the cerebrospinal fluid include all of the following EXCEPT

a. cushioning delicate neurons.

b. supporting peripheral nerves.

c. transporting nutrients to neurons of the brain and cord.

d. removing wastes from the brain and spinal cord.

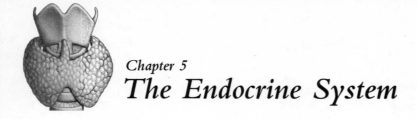

Chapter 5
The Endocrine System

Learning Objectives

- Compare the basic organization and functions of the endocrine and nervous systems.
- Define a hormone, and explain how hormones control their target cells.
- Describe the relationships between the hypothalamus and the pituitary gland.
- Describe the structure and functions of the pituitary gland.
- Describe the manufacture, storage, and secretion of thyroid hormones.
- Describe the function of parathyroid and thymus hormones.
- Describe the structure and functions of the adrenal gland.
- Identify the function of the hormones produced by other endocrine tissues.
- Discuss the results of abnormal hormone production.

Core Concepts

All page references are to the fourth edition of Human Anatomy.

Both the endocrine and nervous systems maintain homeostasis by coordinating the activities of organs and systems throughout the body. The endocrine system is responsible for regulating ongoing processes such as growth and development (page 507). This system includes all the endocrine cells and tissues of the body. Endocrine cells and tissues secrete hormones directly onto their surface or into the blood stream. Hormones can be grouped into four categories based on their chemical structure: amino acid derivatives, peptides, steroids, and eicosanoids (page 508). Hormones influence target cells through receptors located either on the cell membrane or within the cell (page 508).

The hypothalamus regulates activities of both the nervous system and the endocrine system. It does this in three ways: (1) through autonomic centers that exert direct neural control over the endocrine system; (2) by releasing two hormones (ADH and oxytocin); and (3) by secreting regulatory hormones that dictate the activities of endocrine organs (page 509).

The pituitary gland (hypophysis) lies in the sella turcica of the sphenoid (page 510). The posterior lobe (neurohypophysis) contains axons and axon terminals of neurons of the supraoptic and paraventricular nuclei (page 511). These neurons secrete ADH (an anti-diuretic) and oxytocin (a smooth muscle relaxant important in childbirth) as hormones. The anterior lobe of the pituitary gland (adenohypophysis) includes three regions: the pars distalis, the pars intermedia and the pars tuberalis (page 512). The hypophyseal portal system brings regulating hormones from the hypothalamus directly to the anterior lobe of the pituitary gland (page 512). There are seven hormones of the anterior lobe of the pituitary gland (page 512).

Other glands of the endocrine system include the thyroid, parathyroid glands, adrenal glands, thymus, and the reproductive organs (pages 513-521).

The pancreas is both an exocrine and an endocrine gland. The endocrine portion consists of cellular groups called pancreatic islets. These islets are composed of alpha cells, beta cells and F cells, all of which produce their own hormones (page 519).

Labeling Exercise

Label the lettered structures, and then check your answers against the labeled image on the Student Tutor CD.

To locate the image, open your Student Tutor CD by launching the program and clicking **START**. *Use the on-screen navigation menu and click through until you arrive at the* **bold-face** *item indicated.*

Endocrine System > Whole Body

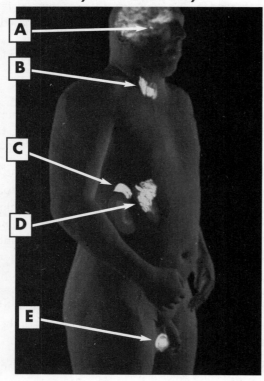

A. _____

B. _____

C. _____

D. _____

E. _____

Scavenger Hunt

This activity offers a unique way for you to familiarize yourself with the location and functions of specific structures.

*Open the Student Tutor CD by launching the program and clicking **START**. Locate the structures displayed in **boldface type** below, and complete the questions that follow.*

1. Left adrenal gland

What structure lies immediately inferior to the left adrenal gland?

What is the function of this lower structure?

2. Pituitary gland

What specific bony structure houses the pituitary gland?

List the nine hormones that are produced by the pituitary gland.

3. Pancreas
Describe the spatial relationship between the pancreas and its nearest endocrine neighbor.

What is unique about the pancreas?

4. Thyroid gland
What hormones are produced by the thyroid gland?

5. Testes
What hormones are produced by the testes and how are they produced?

What endocrine structure governs the production of the hormones of the testes?

6. Parathyroid glands

What hormone is produced by the parathyroid glands and what is its function?

7. Heart

The heart is found in what portion of the thoracic cavity?

What hormones are produced in the heart and what is their function?

Image Comparison

Looking at anatomical structures from many perspectives enables you to learn their general organization and specific structures. By comparing your textbook's illustrations with the 3-dimensional art on the Student Tutor CD, you will sharpen your ability to identify these structures.

Open the Student Tutor CD by launching the program and clicking START. Look at the corresponding images from the CD and textbook listed before each set of questions, then answer the questions.

1. CD: Endocrine System > Glands (rotate 90° to the left)

   Textbook: Figure 19.1

   a. Describe the position of the pituitary gland in relation to the facial features.

   b. How does the pituitary gland control the remaining endocrine glands from its position in the cranial cavity?

2. CD: Endocrine System > Glands (rotate 180° to the right)
   Textbook: Figure 19.9

   a. Describe the structure of the thyroid gland.

   b. Are the parathyroid glands visible on the CD? If so, where do they appear?

3. CD: Endocrine System > Glands (rotate 90° to the right)
   Textbook: Figure 19.10

   a. Describe the physical relationship between the adrenal glands and the kidneys, and the adrenal glands and the pancreas.

Multiple Choice

This section gives you an opportunity to demonstrate your understanding of the material covered in this workbook and in the text. Circle the correct answer for each question.

1. Which of the following is NOT a class of hormones?

   a. small carbohydrates

   b. amino acid derivatives

   c. steroids and eicosanoids

   d. peptide proteins

2. The receptor for thyroid and steroid hormones can be found

   a. on the cell surface.

   b. within the cell membrane.

   c. intracellularly.

   d. extracellularly.

3. The hypothalamus controls the output of the adrenal medullae through

   a. the production of epinephrine and norepinephrine.

   b. the release of regulatory hormones that affect the adrenal medullae.

   c. the production of ADH and oxytocin.

   d. direct control of the sympathetic output via preganglionic fibers.

4. The function of the pars intermedia is

   a. secretion of MSH.

   b. secretion of PRL and GH.

   c. secretion of ADH and oxytocin.

   d. unknown at this time.

5. Growth hormone directly affects the liver, which in turn secretes

   a. somatomedins that stimulate lipid synthesis in the target cells.

   b. somatomedins that stimulate protein synthesis in the target cells.

   c. glucocorticoids that stimulate growth and division of target cells.

   d. mineralocorticoids that stimulate bone growth and development.

6. **The neurons of the paraventricular and supraoptic nuclei of the hypothalamus**

    a. end in the posterior pituitary where they release ADH and oxytocin.

    b. end in the adenohypophysis where they stimulate release of regulating factors.

    c. coordinate functioning of the anterior and posterior lobes of the pituitary.

    d. control the hypophyseal portal system.

7. **The only endocrine gland that stores its hormone product extracellularly is the**

    a. thymus gland.

    b. pancreas.

    c. thyroid gland.

    d. testes.

8. **The C cells of the thyroid produce**

    a. thyroxin.

    b. calcitonin.

    c. Triiodothyronine.

    d. T_4.

9. **Parathyroid hormone is produced by the _____ cells of the parathyroid gland.**

    a. principal

    b. oxyphil

    c. transitional

    d. immature

10. **The zona glomerulosa of the adrenal gland is responsible for the production of**

    a. mineralocorticoids.

    b. glucocorticoids.

    c. aldosterone.

    d. A and C are correct.

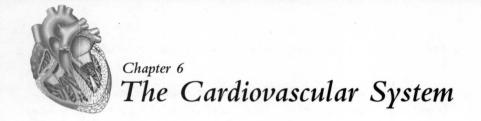

Chapter 6
The Cardiovascular System

Learning Objectives

- List and describe the functions of the blood.
- Discuss the composition of blood and the physical characteristics of plasma.
- List the structural characteristics and functions of the red blood cells.
- Describe the structures and functions of white blood cells.
- Discuss the function of platelets.
- Identify and describe the pericardium, epicardium, and endocardium.
- Identify and describe the external form and surface features of the heart.
- Trace the pathway of blood flow through the heart.
- Locate the coronary blood vessels, their origins, and major branches.
- Describe the general anatomical organization of blood vessels.
- Discuss the various types of blood vessels and their histology.
- Describe the characteristics of capillaries, sinusoids, and capillaries.
- Identify and describe the vessels of the pulmonary circuit.
- Identify the major vessels of the systemic circuit and the areas they supply.

Core Concepts

All page references are to the fourth edition of Human Anatomy.

The cardiovascular system includes the blood, the heart, and the blood vessels of the body. The main function of this system is the transport and exchange of water, solutes, dissolved gases, organic compounds, and blood cells. The fluid used for these exchanges is blood. Blood distributes nutrients, oxygen, and hormones to the cells of the body; it carries metabolic wastes to the kidneys; and it transports specialized cells that defend the body from disease (page 533). Blood is composed of formed elements and plasma. The formed elements are the red blood cells, white blood cells, and platelets (page 533). Plasma differs from interstitial fluid in that it has a higher concentration of dissolved oxygen and a lower concentration of dissolved carbon dioxide than typical interstitial fluid. Plasma also includes dissolved proteins that are not found in interstitial fluid (page 534).

The center of the cardiovascular system is the heart. It lies in the mediastinum, slightly left of the midline, surrounded by a double-walled pericardium (page 550). It sits on an oblique angle to the longitudinal axis of the body, rotated slightly to the left (page 554). There are four chambers to the heart: the left atrium, right atrium, left ventricle, and right ventricle. Papillary muscles, chordae tendineae, and heart valves can be seen within each ventricle (page 557). There are structural differences between the two ventricles (page 558). Valves are found at the junction of the great vessels and within the heart (page 558).

Blood is pumped from the heart through the vessels of the body in the following order: arteries, arterioles, capillaries, venules, and veins (page 573). The structure of the vessel walls changes along this route (page 574). The pulmonary circuit delivers blood to the lungs where oxygen is picked up and carbon dioxide is released (page 580). The systemic circuit begins with blood leaving the heart via the ascending aorta, and ends with blood returning from the body to the heart via the superior and inferior vena cavae (page 580).

Labeling Exercise

Label the lettered structures, and then check your answers against the labeled image on the Student Tutor CD.

To locate the image, open your Student Tutor CD by launching the program and clicking **START**. Use the on-screen navigation menu and click through until you arrive at the **bold-face** item indicated.

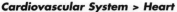

Cardiovascular System > Heart

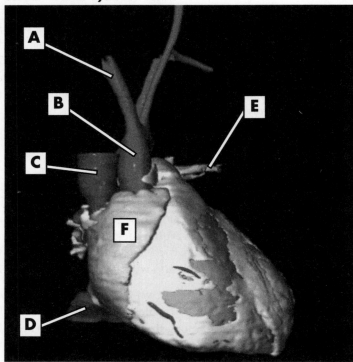

A. _____

B. _____

C. _____

D. _____

E. _____

F. _____

Scavenger Hunt

This activity offers a unique way for you to familiarize yourself with the location and functions of specific structures.

*Open the Student Tutor CD by launching the program and clicking **START**. Locate the structures displayed in **boldface type** below, and complete the questions that follow.*

1. Pulmonary artery

From which ventricle does the pulmonary artery originate?

What tissue, identified on the CD, lies around the base of the pulmonary artery?

2. Superior sagittal sinus

Of what significance is the superior sagittal sinus to the flow of cerebrospinal fluid (CSF)?

Into what major vessel does the superior sagittal sinus drain?

3. Lumbar artery

From which vessel does the lumbar artery directly branch?

What structures are supplied by the lumbar artery?

4. Basilic vein

What is the origin and termination of the basilic vein?

5. Superior (superficial) temporal artery

What structure lies immediately deep to the superior temporal artery?

6. Vertebral artery

Describe the orientation of the vertebral artery.

What structures does the vertebral artery supply?

7. Papillary muscle

In which portion of the heart are the papillary muscles located?

What is attached directly to the papillary muscles?

8. Pulmonary semilunar valve

What two structures are separated by the pulmonary semilunar valve?

9. Superior mesenteric artery

What structures are supplied by the superior mesenteric artery?

Image Comparison

Looking at anatomical structures from many perspectives enables you to learn their general organization and specific structures. By comparing your textbook's illustrations with the 3-dimensional art on the Student Tutor CD, you will sharpen your ability to identify these structures.

Open the Student Tutor CD by launching the program and clicking **START**. *Look at the corresponding images from the CD and textbook listed before each set of questions, then answer the questions.*

1. CD: Cardiovascular System > Upper Limb (second level deep)

Textbook: Figure 22.12

a. What vessels are identical on both presentations?

b. Which vessels are depicted only on the CD?

2. **CD: Cardiovascular System > Lower Extremity**
   Textbook: Figure 22.25

   a. Trace the pathway of the saphenous vein as it courses along the leg and thigh. Which image is more helpful in this task and why?

3. **CD: Cardiovascular System > Abdomen (third layer deep)**
   Textbook: Figure 22.26

   a. Trace the veins originating from the capillary beds of the superior and inferior mesenteric veins. How do these veins function in comparison to veins of the lower limb?

Multiple Choice

This section gives you an opportunity to demonstrate your understanding of the material covered in this workbook and in the text. Circle the correct answer for each question.

1. The blood cell responsible for specific immunity is the

    a. neutrophil.

    b. eosinophil.

    c. lymphocyte.

    d. erythrocyte.

2. The function of the platelets is to

    a. carry oxygen to tissues.

    b. remove carbon dioxide from tissues.

    c. protect the body from pathogens.

    d. help prevent fluid loss.

3. The innermost layer of the heart wall is the

    a. myocardium.

    b. epicardium.

    c. endocardium.

    d. pericardium.

4. The valve that prevents backflow of blood from the right ventricle to the right atrium is the

    a. tricuspid valve.

    b. bicuspid valve.

    c. mitral valve.

    d. pulmonary semilunar valve.

5. The first pair of arteries to branch off the aorta are the

    a. subclavians.

    b. brachial arteries.

    c. coronary arteries.

    d. axillary arteries.

6. Which of the following is NOT an artery of the arm?

  a. axillary artery

  b. thoracocervical artery

  c. deep brachial artery

  d. humoral circumflex artery

7. The subclavian artery is called the _____ artery after it passes distally from beneath the clavicle.

  a. brachial

  b. radial

  c. axillary

  d. humeral circumflex

8. The abdominal aorta branches at its end into the

  a. common iliac arteries.

  b. left and right femoral arteries.

  c. left and right lumbar arteries.

  d. external and internal iliac arteries.

9. The genicular arteries are found surrounding the

  a. upper femur.

  b. lateral ankle region.

  c. knee.

  d. quadriceps muscle group.

10. The sinuses of the brain all drain into the

  a. vertebral artery.

  b. external jugular vein.

  c. brachiocephalic vein.

  d. internal jugular vein.

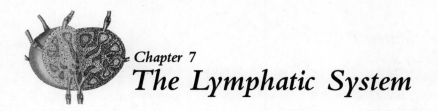

Chapter 7
The Lymphatic System

Learning Objectives

- Describe the role played by the lymphatic system in the body's defenses.
- Identify the major components of the lymphatic system.
- Contrast the structure of lymphatic vessels and veins.
- Describe the location, structure, and function of lymphatic vessels.
- Describe the anatomical and functional relationship between the lymphatic and cardiovascular systems.
- Describe the location and function of the thymus, lymph nodes, and spleen.

Core Concepts

All page references are to the fourth edition of Human Anatomy.

The human body has several defense mechanisms against injury and disease. The lymphatic system, interacting with other systems of the body, provides a strong defense against invading pathogens. The lymphatic system is composed of a network of lymphatic vessels, fluid within these vessels (lymph), and lymphoid tissues and organs which monitor and alter the composition of the lymph (page 613). The functions of the lymphatic system include: the production, maintenance, and distribution of lymphocytes; the maintenance of normal blood volume and the elimination of local variations in the chemical composition of interstitial fluid; and the provision of an alternative route for the transport of hormones, nutrients, and waste products (page 613).

Lymphatic vessels are similar to veins, except they are part of an open system. There is no circuit of vessels for lymph. Lymph is picked up by lymphatic capillaries, or terminal capillaries, from within tissues. Lymphatic capillaries differ from vascular capillaries in that: 1) they are larger in diameter and sectional view; 2) they have thinner walls; 3) they have flat or irregular outlines; and 4) the endothelial cells of the walls overlap forming one-way valves for the entrance of fluid (page 615). Lymphatic vessels have valves to prevent backflow (page 615). Pressure within the lymphatic vessels is extremely low, and lymph is moved along by compression of the vessels during skeletal muscle movement and breathing (page 616).

Lymphocytes are the major cells of the lymphatic system. There are three different classes of lymphocytes: T-cells, B-cells, and NK cells (page 617). Lymphoid tissues are connective tissues dominated by lymphocytes. Lymphoid nodules are found in the respiratory, digestive, urinary, and reproductive systems.

Labeling Exercise #1

The lymphatic system is an intricate connection of lymphatic vessels, lymph nodes, and lymphoid organs. Upon completing the labeling exercise below, continue to the next page with a "View & Compare" activity.

Lymphatic System (Figure 23.1)

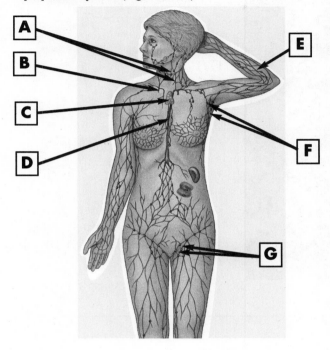

A. _____

B. _____

C. _____

D. _____

E. _____

F. _____

G. _____

Labeling Exercise #2 - View & Compare

Locate the image on your CD as pictured below, then open your textbook to page 613 to view Figure 23.1. On the diagrams below, draw a line to the structures that are depicted on BOTH the CD and in Figure 23.1, adding lettered labels as in Labeling Exercise #1. (Be sure to manipulate the image on your CD to obtain all possible angles.) Write out these structures on the lines provided.

Lymphatic System > Whole Body

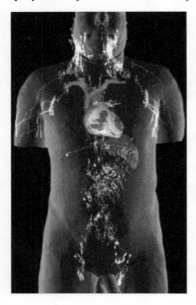

Figure 23.1

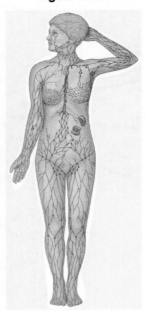

_____

_____

_____

_____

_____

_____

_____

_____

Scavenger Hunt

This activity offers a unique way for you to familiarize yourself with the location and functions of specific structures.

Open the Student Tutor CD by launching the program and clicking **START**. *Locate the structures displayed in* **boldface type** *below, and complete the questions that follow.*

1. Spleen

What lymphatic nodes lie closest to the spleen?

Using what you know of the anatomy of the spleen and the organs of the abdominal cavity, what organs surround the spleen?

2. Left axillary nodes

Can you palpate the left axillary on a healthy human body?
Explain your answer.

What might a swollen lymph node in this region indicate?

3. Tracheal nodes

What system is protected by the activity of the tracheal nodes?

What type of pathogen would you expect these to combat?

4. Pancreatic nodes

What organ lies immediately superior to the pancreas?

Is there any lymphatic tissue shown in that organ? If so, what label is given to that lymphatic tissue?

5. Thoracic duct

What is the function of the thoracic duct?

What lies immediately anterior to the thoracic duct?

6. Spinal accessory nodes

The spinal accesory nodes an important immunological role for what region of the body?

What other lymph nodes are present in the same area?

Image Comparison

Looking at anatomical structures from many perspectives enables you to learn their general organization and specific structures. By comparing your textbook's illustrations with the 3-dimensional art on the Student Tutor CD, you will sharpen your ability to identify these structures.

Open the Student Tutor CD by launching the program and clicking START. Look at the corresponding images from the CD and textbook listed before each set of questions, then answer the questions.

1. CD: Lymphatic System > Whole Body

   Textbook: Figure 23.11

   a. How does the lymphatic drainage of the pectoral region differ between males and females?

2. CD: Lymphatic System > Whole Body

   Textbook: Figure 23.13

   a. Compare the CD depiction of the inguinal lymph nodes with that of the pelvic lymphangiogram. What structures are these lymph nodes and lymphatic ducts following as they lay in the inguinal region?

b. Of what medical benefit is the lymphangiogram?

3. CD: Lymphatic System > Whole Body (rotate 90° to the right)
   Textbook: Figure 23.17

   a. Describe the location of the spleen in relation to the lymph glands of the
      abdominal cavity. What structures lie adjacent to the spleen?

Multiple Choice

This section gives you an opportunity to demonstrate your understanding of the material covered in this workbook and in the text. Circle the correct answer for each question.

1. The functions of the lymphatic system include all of the following EXCEPT

    a. maintenance of interstitial fluid pH.

    b. provision of a route for hormone delivery.

    c. production and maintenance of populations of lymphocytes.

    d. maintenance of normal blood volume.

2. Lymphatic vessels differ from vascular vessels in that

    a. lymphatic vessels have valves, while vascular vessels do not.

    b. lymphatic vessel walls are thicker than vascular vessel walls.

    c. lymphatic capillaries have loosely connected endothelial cells.

    d. both A and B are correct.

3. Which of the following structures would be found at the origin of the thoracic duct?

    a. right lymphatic vessel

    b. thoracic terminus

    c. heart

    d. cisterna chyli

4. The _____ collects lymph from both sides of the body inferior to the diaphragm and from the left side of the body superior to the diaphragm.

    a. thoracic duct

    b. right lymphatic duct

    c. superficial lymphatics

    d. deep lymphatics

5. Lymph nodes include _____ entrance(s) and _____ exit(s).

    a. one; many

    b. many; one

    c. one; one

    d. many; many

6. The _____ lymph nodes filter fluid coming from the urinary and reproductive systems.

a. abdominal

b. mesenterial

c. popliteal

d. axillary

7. The thymic hormones are produced by the

a. red pulp of the thymus.

b. epithelial cells of the thymus.

c. white pulp of the thymus.

d. lymphocytes within the thymus.

8. Examples of lymphoid tissue include all of the following EXCEPT

a. tonsils.

b. MALT.

c. spleen.

d. aggregated nodules.

9. Antibody mediated immunity is carried out by

a. B cells.

b. cytotoxic T cells.

c. helper T cells.

d. suppressor T cells.

10. Lymph originating from the intestines is picked up and filtered through the

a. mesenterial lymph nodes.

b. intestinal lymph nodes.

c. aggregated lymphoid nodules.

d. all of the above.

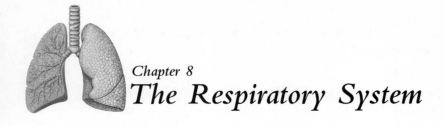

Chapter 8
The Respiratory System

Learning Objectives

- Describe the primary functions of the respiratory system.
- Describe the structural organization of the respiratory system and its major organs.
- Distinguish between the conducting and respiratory portions of the respiratory tract.
- Describe the functional anatomy of the components of the upper respiratory tract.
- Describe the functional anatomy of the larynx.
- Discuss the gross anatomical specializations of the trachea.
- Describe the functional anatomy of the bronchial tree and bronchopulmonary segments.
- Describe the structure and function of the respiratory membrane.
- Describe the pleural cavities and pleural membranes.
- Identify the muscles of respiration.

Core Concepts

All page references are to the fourth edition of Human Anatomy.

The respiratory system is responsible for facilitating the movement of oxygen to the cells of the body, removing carbon dioxide from the cells of the body, and assisting in the regulation of the body's blood pressure, blood volume, and pH. The organs of the respiratory system include the nose, nasal cavity and sinuses, the pharynx, larynx, trachea, and the smaller conducting passageways leading to the gas-exchange surfaces of the lungs (page 635).

The nose and nasal cavity are the primary passageways for air entering the respiratory system. The external nares open to the environment. They lead into the vestibule, separated into left and right halves by the nasal septum (page 637). The turbinate bones project toward the nasal septum from the lateral walls of the nasal cavity, and assist in swirling the incoming air through the nasal cavity. Air then moves into the pharynx, which has shared digestive and respiratory functions. It is divided into the nasopharynx, oropharynx, and laryngopharynx (page 637).

The larynx serves as the divider between the upper and lower respiratory tract. The larynx contains three large unpaired cartilages and three smaller paired cartilages (pages 639–640). Ligaments of the larynx include the intrinsic ligaments, the extrinsic ligaments, and the vestibular ligaments (page 641). Intrinsic and extrinsic laryngeal musculature regulate tension in the vocal folds, as well as positioning and stabilizing the larynx (page 641).

The trachea, or windpipe, extends from the larynx to the lungs. At the end of the trachea lies the left and right primary bronchi, which enter the lungs at the hilus. The primary bronchi branch, forming the bronchial tree (pages 642–648). The right primary bronchus branches into the superior lobar bronchus, a middle lobar bronchus, and an inferior lobar bronchus. The left primary bronchus divides into two secondary bronchi, a superior bronchus, and an inferior bronchus (page 645). These bronchi then branch into terminal bronchioles, which lead into a single pulmonary lobule. Each lobule is fed by several delicate respiratory bronchioles (page 648), which are connected to the alveolar sacs via alveolar ducts (page 648). The respiratory membrane includes simple squamous epithelium, septal cells, and alveolar macrophages (page 648).

Each lung lies in a pleural cavity lined by a serous membrane called the pleura. The parietal pleura covers the inner surface of the thoracic cavity, while the visceral pleura covers the outer surface of the lungs (page 651). Pulmonary ventilation refers to the physical movement of air into and out of the lungs. It is accomplished by the diaphragm, and the external and internal intercostal muscles (page 654). Accessory respiratory muscles are used when increasing the depth or frequency of respirations.

Labeling Exercise

Label the lettered structures, and then check your answers against the labeled image on the
Student Tutor CD.

To locate the image, open your Student Tutor CD by launching the program and clicking
START. Use the on-screen navigation menu and click through until you arrive at the **boldface** item indicated.

Respiratory System > Lungs

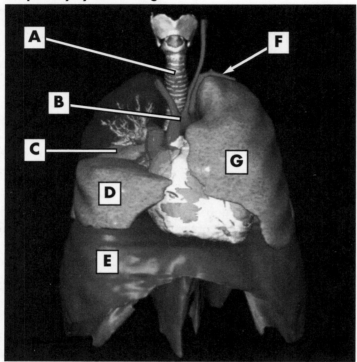

A. _____

B. _____

C. _____

D. _____

E. _____

F. _____

G. _____

Scavenger Hunt

This activity offers a unique way for you to familiarize yourself with the location and functions of specific structures.

Open the Student Tutor CD by launching the program and clicking **START**. *Locate the structures displayed in* **boldface type** *below, and complete the questions that follow.*

1. Anular ligaments of trachea

What is the function of the anular ligaments?

Describe the shape of the cartilage above and below these rings.

2. Arytenoid cartilage

What cartilage lies anterior to the arytenoid cartilage in the larynx, and upon what cartilage is this supported?

What is the function of the arytenoid cartilage?

3. Left inferior lobe of the lungs

Describe the location of the left inferior lobe of the lungs.

What portion of the heart is closest to this lobe?

4. Diaphragm

Describe the shape of the diaphragm.

Using what you know of general anatomy, what structures lie inferior to the diaphragm, causing the shape seen?

5. Superior lobar bronchus

Trace the respiratory pathway from the nasal cavity to the superior lobar bronchus.

6. Pulmonary artery

What structure follows the pathway of the pulmonary artery?

What is the function of this artery?

Image Comparison

Looking at anatomical structures from many perspectives enables you to learn their general organization and specific structures. By comparing your textbook's illustrations with the 3-dimensional art on the Student Tutor CD, you will sharpen your ability to identify these structures.

*Open the Student Tutor CD by launching the program and clicking **START**. Look at the corresponding images from the CD and textbook listed before each set of questions, then answer the questions.*

1. **CD: Respiratory System > Lungs**
   Textbook: Figure 24.8

   a. Describe the location and appearance of the left lung. Does it appear similar on both the CD and in the book?

2. **CD: Respiratory System > Lungs (seventh level deep)**
   Textbook: Figure 24.10

   a. Where does the heart lie in relation to the left inferior lobar bronchus?

   b. Which lung has the longer bronchial tree?

3. **CD: Respiratory System > Lung Flythrough (trachial cut-away and respiratory epithelium in view)**
   Textbook: Figure 24.2

   a. What function do the goblet cells have in the respiratory epithelium?

   b. In which direction do the cilia of the respiratory epithelium push the overlying mucus?

4. **CD: Respiratory System > Lung Flythrough (second histological enlargement in view, at the alveolar sac)**
   Textbook: Figure 24.12

   a. What cells make up the respiratory membrane?

   b. Describe the internal appearance of the alveolar sac.

Multiple Choice

This section gives you an opportunity to demonstrate your understanding of the material covered in this workbook and in the text. Circle the correct answer for each question.

1. The respiratory epithelium consists of

    a. pseudostratified ciliated columnar epithelium.

    b. pseudostratified columnar epithelium.

    c. goblet cells.

    d. pseudostratified ciliated columnar epithelium and goblet cells.

2. The structures of the oropharynx include all of the following EXCEPT

    a. the palatine tonsils.

    b. the fauces.

    c. the uvula.

    d. the pharyngeal tonsil.

3. The _____ cartilage of the larynx is involved with the opening and closing of the glottis and the production of sound.

    a. corniculate

    b. epiglottis

    c. thyroid

    d. arytenoid

4. The right lung includes all of the following EXCEPT

    a. a middle lobe.

    b. a cardiac notch.

    c. a lower lobe.

    d. a root.

5. The correct sequence of intrapulmonary bronchi is

    a. tertiary bronchi > lobar bronchi > segmental bronchi

    b. primary bronchi > lobar bronchi > segmental bronchi

    c. segmental bronchi > primary bronchi > lobar bronchi

    d. primary bronchi > segmental bronchi > lobar bronchi

6. In the respiratory system, sympathetic activation leads to

a. excess mucus production

b. bronchodilation

c. excess surfactant production

d. bronchoconstriction

7. Type I cells, or respiratory epitheliocytes, are usually

a. extremely thin.

b. quite robust.

c. lined with cilia.

d. dotted with pores.

8. Surfactant

a. patrols epithelium by removing pathogens.

b. provides moisture for gas exchange.

c. carries oxygen across the respiratory membrane.

d. reduces surface tension in the fluid coating the alveoli.

9. The conducting portion of the respiratory system extends from

a. the entrance to the nasal cavities to the larynx.

b. the entrance to the nasal cavities to the trachea.

c. the entrance to the nasal cavities to the terminal bronchioles.

d. the entrance to the nasal cavities to the respiratory bronchioles.

10. Hyperpnea is defined as

a. quiet breathing.

b. costal breathing.

c. forced breathing.

d. deep breathing.

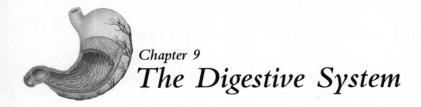

Chapter 9
The Digestive System

Learning Objectives

- Summarize the functions of the digestive system.
- Locate the components of the digestive tract and accessory organs, and state their functions.
- Describe the peritoneum and the locations and functions of the mesenteries.
- Describe the gross and microscopic structure of the tongue, teeth, and salivary glands.
- Describe the general structure and function of the pharynx.
- Describe the anatomy of the stomach, its functions and its regulatory hormones.
- Describe the anatomy of the small and large intestine and their regulatory hormones.
- Describe the anatomy of the liver and gall bladder.
- Describe the anatomy of the pancreas and the hormones that regulate it.
- Describe the changes in the digestive system that occur with aging.

Core Concepts

All page references are to the fourth edition of Human Anatomy.

The digestive system consists of the digestive tract and various accessory organs. The oral cavity, pharynx, esophagus, stomach, small intestine, and large intestine make up the digestive tract. Accessory digestive organs include the teeth and tongue, along with glandular organs such as the salivary glands, liver, and pancreas (page 663). The functions of the digestive tract and accessory organs are: ingestion, mechanical processing, digestion, secretion, absorption, compaction, and excretion (page 663).

The visceral peritoneum and the parietal peritoneum line the abdominal cavity. Sheets of serous membrane, the mesenteries, connect the two layers of the peritoneum and suspend the digestive tract (page 667). The mesenteries include the lesser and greater omentum, the mesentery proper, and the mesocolon (page 667).

The first area of the digestive tract is the oral cavity. The oral cavity is composed of oral mucosa, labia, cheeks, vestibule, gingivae, hard and soft palates, the uvula, tongue, and teeth (page 667). The parotid, sublingual and submandibular salivary glands are also found in the oral cavity (page 672). There are four types of teeth that assist in mechanical digestion: incisors, cuspids, bicuspids, and molars (page 673).

The pharynx is a shared passageway for both the digestive and respiratory systems. The esophagus is the hollow muscular tube through which the bolus of food travels to reach the stomach (page 676). The stomach has three major functions: bulk storage of ingested material, mechanical breakdown of ingested material, and chemical digestion of ingested material through acids and enzymes (page 677). The small intestine digests and absorbs nutrients. The regions of the small intestine include the duodenum, the jejunum, and the ileum (page 683). The small intestine is held in place by the mesentery proper (page 683). The large intestine has five sections: the cecum, ascending colon, transverse colon, descending colon, and sigmoid colon (page 686). The rectum forms the end of the digestive tract. Accessory organs of the digestive system include the liver, salivary glands, gall bladder, and pancreas. The liver is the largest visceral organ (page 689). The liver has four lobes: the right, left, caudate, and quadrate lobes (page 690). Two blood vessels deliver blood to the liver: the hepatic artery and the hepatic portal vein. Bile is secreted by the liver, and it is stored and modified in the gall bladder (page 692).

The gall bladder lies on the ventral surface of the right lobe of the liver (page 693). Bile is released through the common bile duct into the duodenum. The pancreas, which has a head, body and tail (page 693) is primarily an exocrine gland, secreting digestive enzymes through the pancreatic duct into the duodenum (page 694).

Labeling Exercise #1

Label the lettered structures, and then check your answers against the labeled image on the Student Tutor CD.

*To locate the images in the exercises that follow, open your Student Tutor CD by launching the program and clicking **START**. Use the on-screen navigation menu and click through until you arrive at the **boldface** item indicated.*

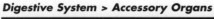

Digestive System > Accessory Organs

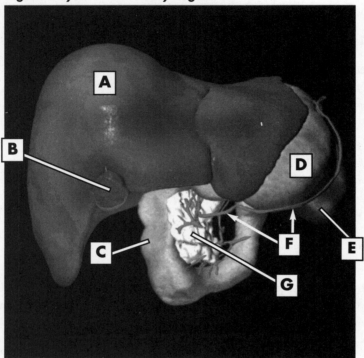

A. _____

B. _____

C. _____

D. _____

E. _____

F. _____

G. _____

Labeling Exercise #2

Digestive System > Digestive

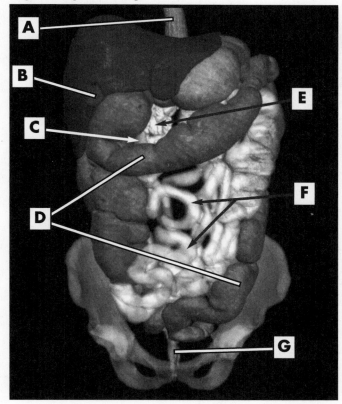

A. _____

B. _____

C. _____

D. _____

E. _____

F. _____

G. _____

Scavenger Hunt

This activity offers a unique way for you to familiarize yourself with the location and functions of specific structures.

*Open the Student Tutor CD by launching the program and clicking **START**. Locate the structures displayed in **boldface type** below, and complete the questions that follow.*

1. Greater omentum

Where is the origin of the greater omentum?

What is the function of this structure?

2. Hepatic ducts of quadrate lobe

Describe the position of the quadrate lobe.

What fluid is carried in the hepatic ducts?

3. Pancreatic duct

What is carried in the pancreatic duct?

4. Small intestine

What portion of the small intestine lies within the pelvic cavity?

5. Gastric artery

What other structure of the digestive system does the gastric artery travel across to reach the stomach?

Identify the artery that travels deep to the gastric artery, and runs to the right rather than straight up to the stomach.

Image Comparison

Looking at anatomical structures from many perspectives enables you to learn their general organization and specific structures. By comparing your textbook's illustrations with the 3-dimensional art on the Student Tutor CD, you will sharpen your ability to identify these structures.

*Open the Student Tutor CD by launching the program and clicking **START**. Look at the corresponding images from the CD and textbook listed before each set of questions, then answer the questions.*

1. **CD: Digestive System > Accessory Organs**
   Textbook: Figure 25.23

   a. What differences do you see in the pathway of the arteries presented on the CD when compared to the text diagram?

   b. How does the pancreaticoduodenal artery compare in the two images?

2. **CD: Digestive System > Digestive (third level deep)**
   Textbook: Figure 25.1

   a. Where does the transverse colon lie with respect to the stomach, and what accessory organs lie close to the transverse colon?

3. CD: Digestive System > Digestive (fourth level deep)
   Textbook: Figure 25.18

   a. Which depiction provides more information concerning the shape and pathway of the colon?

4. CD: Digestive System > Mastication movie (last portion)
   Textbook: Figure 25.3

   a. What organ initiates the peristaltic wave that pushes food through the digestive tract?

   b. How does the bolus get directed into the esophagus from the pharynx?

Multiple Choice

This section gives you an opportunity to demonstrate your understanding of the material covered in this workbook and in the text. Circle the correct answer for each question.

1. The correct order for the four major layers of the digestive tract is

   a. submucosa > muscularis > mucosa > serosa.

   b. serosa > mucosa > muscularis > submucosa.

   c. mucosa > submucosa > muscularis > serosa.

   d. mucosa > submucosa > serosa > muscularis.

2. The organs that are retroperitoneal include

   a. the stomach and the duodenum.

   b. the pancreas and duodenum.

   c. the ascending and descending colon.

   d. both B and C are correct.

3. The _____ phase of swallowing involves elevation of the larynx and reflection of the epiglottis.

   a. pharyngeal

   b. buccal

   c. esophageal

   d. laryngeal

4. The chief cells of the gastric pits secrete

   a. gastrin.

   b. pepsinogen.

   c. intrinsic factor.

   d. pepsin.

5. Functions of the stomach include

   a. bulk storage and enzymatic lipid digestion.

   b. enzymatic lipid digestion and mechanical processing.

   c. enzymatic carbohydrate digestion and bulk storage.

   d. bulk storage and mechanical processing.

6. **Lacteals are found in the**

    a. rugae of the stomach.
    b. villi of the small intestine.
    c. haustra of the large intestine.
    d. plicae of the small intestine.

7. **The vermiform appendix is attached to the**

    a. cecum.
    b. ascending colon.
    c. transverse colon.
    d. ileocecal valve.

8. **Compared to the small intestine, the large intestine has**

    a. thicker walls and a smaller diameter.
    b. thicker walls and a larger diameter.
    c. thinner walls and a smaller diameter.
    d. thinner walls and a larger diameter.

9. **The lobe of the liver that houses the gall bladder is the**

    a. left lobe.
    b. right lobe.
    c. caudate lobe.
    d. quadrate lobe.

10. **The portion of the pancreas that secretes digestive enzymes is the**

    a. pancreatic islets.
    b. pancreatic head.
    c. pancreatic acini.
    d. pancreatic juice.

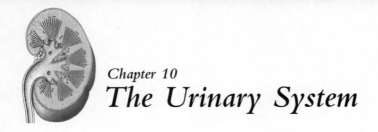

Chapter 10
The Urinary System

Learning Objectives

- Describe the functions of the urinary system.
- Identify the components of the urinary system and their functions.
- Identify the structure and function of each anatomical feature of the kidneys.
- Describe the location of the kidneys, their external features, and their relationship to adjacent tissues and organs.
- Identify the blood vessels that supply the nephrons.
- Describe the unusual characteristics and properties of glomerular capillaries.
- Describe the organization of the nephron and the functions of each segment.
- Describe the location and gross anatomy of the ureters, urinary bladder, and urethra.
- Discuss the micturition reflex and its control.

Core Concepts

All page references are to the fourth edition of Human Anatomy.

The functions of the urinary system include: 1) regulating plasma concentrations of sodium, potassium, chloride, calcium, and other ions; 2) regulating blood volume and blood pressure; 3) contributing to the stabilization of blood pH; 4) conserving valuable nutrients; 5) eliminating organic waste products; 6) synthesizing calcitriol; and 7) assisting the liver (page 703). The organs responsible for this list of functions are the kidneys, ureters, urinary bladder, and urethra.

The kidneys are retroperitoneal. They are covered by a renal capsule and protected by an adipose tissue capsule (page 703). The blood vessels and lymphatics of the kidney enter at the hilus (page 704). Blood supply to the kidneys flows from a renal artery through segmental arteries, interlobar arteries, arcuate arteries, interlobular arteries, afferent arterioles, and efferent arterioles. Venous return follows the same pattern, although there are no segmental veins (page 707).

Within the kidney there are three distinct areas: the cortex, medulla, and pelvis (page 703). Urine is produced by microscopic nephrons found within the cortex and medulla of each kidney (page 705). The nephron is the functional unit of the urinary system. It is responsible for blood filtration and maintenance of ion concentrations (pages 708–712). The collecting system of the kidney then collects the finely tuned waste urine, making final adjustments in osmotic concentration and volume (page 712).

The ureters, urinary bladder, and urethra transport, store, and eliminate waste. The ureters are muscular tubes that extend from the pelvis of the kidney to the ureteral opening of the urinary bladder (page 714). The urinary bladder is a hollow muscular organ lined with transitional epithelium (page 714). The base of the urinary bladder is the trigone, formed by the ureteral openings and the entrance to the urethra (page 714). The urethra extends from the neck of the bladder to the exterior. It varies in length based on gender (page 714). Micturition is controlled at the urethra by the control of the external urethral sphincter (page 717).

Labeling Exercise

Label the lettered structures, and then check your answers against the labeled image on the Student Tutor CD.

To locate the image, open your Student Tutor CD by launching the program and clicking **START**. Use the on-screen navigation menu and click through until you arrive at the **bold-face** item indicated.

Urinary System > Male Dissection (second level deep, posterior view)

A. _____

B. _____

C. _____

D. _____

E. _____

Scavenger Hunt

This activity offers a unique way for you to familiarize yourself with the location and functions of specific structures.

*Open the Student Tutor CD by launching the program and clicking **START**. Locate the structures displayed in **bold-faced type** below, and complete the questions that follow.*

1. Urethra

What structure(s) of the reproductive system lie adjacent to the urethra in the male?

Which is responsible for problems with the micturition reflex in aging males?

2. Left kidney

Why is the left kidney not found at the same lumbar level as the right kidney?

3. Ureter

Describe the pathway of the ureters from the kidneys to the bladder.

What structures of the pelvic and abdominal cavities are found in close proximity to the ureters?

4. Urinary bladder

Describe the general shape of the urinary bladder.

What structure might be responsible for the shape of the anterior surface of the bladder?

Image Comparison

Looking at anatomical structures from many perspectives enables you to learn their general organization and specific structures. By comparing your textbook's illustrations with the 3-dimensional art on the Student Tutor CD, you will sharpen your ability to identify these structures.

Open the Student Tutor CD by launching the program and clicking START. Look at the corresponding images from the CD and textbook listed before each set of questions, then answer the questions.

1. **CD: Urinary System > Dissection > Male**
   Textbook: Figure 26.1, Part A

   a. What structural differences are there between the male and female urinary system? Compare each of the related organs individually.

   b. Define the boundaries of the space the urinary bladder occupies in the pelvic cavity.

2. CD: Urinary System > Male Flythrough (seventh screen)
   Textbook: Figure 26.3

   a. Through which structures does the filtrate travel as it is processed into urine? List, in order, the portions of the nephron and collecting system through which filtrate travels as it is processed into urine.

3. CD: Urinary System > Male Flythrough (last screen, before "click to continue" command)
   Textbook: Figure 26.10

   a. Describe the internal structure of the urinary bladder. Is there a visible difference in the inner wall of the bladder at the trigone?

Multiple Choice

This section gives you an opportunity to demonstrate your understanding of the material covered in this workbook and in the text. Circle the correct answer for each question.

1. The functions of the urinary system include all of the following EXCEPT

    a. contributing to the stabilization of blood pH.

    b. regulating blood concentrations of glucose.

    c. synthesizing calcitriol.

    d. assisting the liver in detoxification.

2. The position of the kidneys is maintained by

    a. the peritoneum.

    b. adjacent visceral organs.

    c. supporting connective tissues.

    d. all of the above.

3. The portion of the kidneys that includes the renal pyramids is the

    a. medulla.

    b. cortex.

    c. pelvis.

    d. hilum.

4. The correct sequence of arteries through which renal blood flows is

    a. interlobular artery > interlobar artery > arcuate artery > afferent arteriole.

    b. segmental artery > afferent arteriole > arcuate artery > interlobar artery.

    c. segmental artery > interlobar artery > arcuate artery > interlobular artery.

    d. interlobular artery > segmental artery > interlobar artery > arcuate artery.

5. The portion of the nephron responsible for collecting the filtrate is the

    a. PCT.

    b. renal corpuscle.

    c. DCT.

    d. Loop of Henle.

6. Which of the following is responsible for the filtration slits in the renal corpuscle?

   a. podocytes
   b. capillary endothelium
   c. basement membrane
   d. capsular space

7. The paired structures used during urine transport, storage, and elimination are individually referred to as the

   a. ureter.
   b. urethra.
   c. urinary bladder.
   d. adrenal gland.

8. The osseous support for the urinary bladder includes the

   a. ischium.
   b. ilium.
   c. pubis.
   d. all of the above.

9. The male urethra passes through the

   a. corpora cavernosa.
   b. corpus spongiosum.
   c. prostate gland.
   d. B and C are correct.

10. The longest tube in the female urinary system is the

   a. urethra.
   b. ureter.
   c. PCT.
   d. collecting tubule.

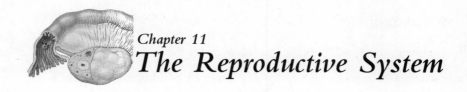

Chapter 11
The Reproductive System

Learning Objectives

- Describe the function of the reproductive system.
- Compare the organization of the male and female reproductive systems.
- Describe the location, gross anatomy, and functions of the male reproductive structures.
- Trace the path of sperm following spermiogenesis.
- Discuss the storage and transport of sperm cells and the components of semen.
- Describe the location, gross anatomy, and functions of the female reproductive structures.
- Trace the path of oocytes following ovulation.

Core Concepts

All page references are to the fourth edition of Human Anatomy.

The function of the reproductive system is to produce, nourish, and transport functional male and female gametes (page 725). There are two functionally and anatomically distinct reproductive systems: the male system and the female system.

The male reproductive system includes the testes, epididymus, ductus deferens, seminal vesicles, ejaculatory duct, prostate gland, bulbourethral glands, urethra, penis, and scrotum (page 726). The testes are the sites of sperm production and are composed of tightly coiled seminiferous tubules held within lobules (page 728). The seminiferous tubules connect to the rete testis which in turn connects to the epididymis (page 729). Spermatogenesis occurs within the seminiferous tubules (page 729). Spermatids mature into sperm (spermiogenesis) within the sustentacular cells of the seminiferous tubules (pages 729–731). The functions of the epididymis include monitoring and adjusting the composition of the fluid from the seminiferous tubules, recycling damaged spermatozoa, storing spermatozoa and facilitating their maturation (page 732). The ductus deferens connects the epididymis to the ejaculatory duct. Sperm travels through the inguinal canal within the ductus deferens as part of the spermatic cord (page 732). The sperm travel next through the urethra (page 732), and out of the body via the penis. The accessory glands of the male reproductive system include the seminal vesicles, the prostate gland, and the bulbourethral glands (pages 733–735).

The female reproductive system consists of paired ovaries and uterine tubes, the uterus, vagina, and the external genitalia (page 737). The ovaries are small paired organs held in place in the abdominal cavity by the ovarian and suspensory ligaments (page 737). Oogenesis occurs in the ovary under the influence of FHS (page 740). Ovulation occurs under the influence of LH (page 741). The structural support for the remaining follicle develops into the corpus luteum, which then degenerates into the corpus albicans (page 741). The ovulated egg is picked up by the uterine tubes (page 742). The uterus provides mechanical protection, nutritional support, and waste removal for a developing fetus (page 743). The uterus has a body, fundus, isthmus, and cervix (page 743). The uterine wall is composed of an outer incomplete lining, the perimetrium, and a middle muscular myometrium lined internally with endometrium (page 744). The endometrium undergoes monthly changes directed by hormones (page 746). The vagina or birth canal is a muscular tube extending from the cervix of the uterus to the vestibule of external genitalia (page 747). The external genitalia of the female is called the vulva. It includes the labia minora, paraurethral glands, clitoris and prepuce (page 749). The mammary glands lie on either side of the chest, in the pectoral fat pad deep to the skin. These are composed of glandular tissue arranged in lobules, and a lactiferous sinus that drains through a nipple in the areola (page 749). Suspensory ligaments of the breast hold this tissue in place (page 750).

Labeling Exercise #1

Label the lettered structures, and then check your answers against the labeled image on the Student Tutor CD.

To locate the images in the exercises that follow, open your Student Tutor CD by launching the program and clicking **START**. Use the on-screen navigation menu and click through until you arrive at the **boldface** item indicated.

Reproductive System > Female Dissection

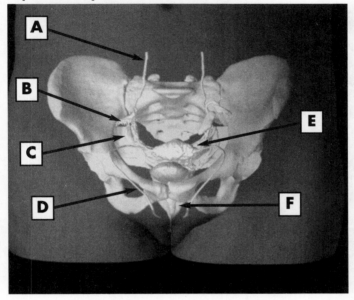

A. _____

B. _____

C. _____

D. _____

E. _____

F. _____

Labeling Exercise #2

Reproductive System > Male Dissection (second layer deep)

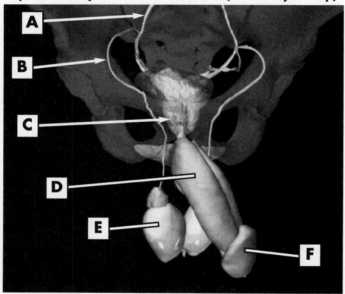

A. _____

B. _____

C. _____

D. _____

E. _____

F. _____

Scavenger Hunt

This activity offers a unique way for you to familiarize yourself with the location and functions of specific structures.

Open the Student Tutor CD by launching the program and clicking **START**. *Locate the structures displayed in* **boldface type** *below, and complete the questions that follow.*

1. Broad ligament

What structure is held in place by the broad ligament?

2. Right ovary

What structures are found surrounding the right ovary?

3. Epididymis

Describe the position of the head, body, and tail of the epididymis in relation to the testicle.

4. Corpus spongiosum

What structure lies in the center of the corpus spongiosum?

5. Ductus deferens

What structures does the ductus deferens connect? Describe its location in relation to the inguinal canal and the urinary bladder.

6. Bulbourethral gland

What is the function of the bulbourethral gland?

How is the location of the bulbourethral gland related to its name?

7. Uterus

Describe the placement of the uterus in relation to the broad ligament.

What is the relationship between the uterus and the urinary bladder?

Image Comparison

Looking at anatomical structures from many perspectives enables you to learn their general organization and specific structures. By comparing your textbook's illustrations with the 3-dimensional art on the Student Tutor CD, you will sharpen your ability to identify these structures.

Open the Student Tutor CD by launching the program and clicking START. Look at the corresponding images from the CD and textbook listed before each set of questions, then answer the questions.

1. **CD: Reproductive System > Male Dissection (rotate 180°)**
   Textbook: Figure 27.1, Part I

   a. Describe the relationship between the ureters and the ductus deferens. Which view makes this easier to visualize?

2. **CD: Reproductive System > Male Dissection (second level deep, rotate 90° clockwise)**
   Textbook: Figure 27.9c

   a. Describe the relationship between the corpora cavernosa and the corpus spongiosum.

b. Which figure provides more useful information about the relationship between these structures? Explain.

3. CD: Reproductive System > Male Flythrough
Textbook: Figure 27.5

a. How does the animation compare with the succession of figures in the text beginning with Figure 27.5 and ending with Figure 27.6? What is the best presentation of the entire process? Explain.

4. CD: Reproductive System > Female Dissection (second level deep)
   Textbook: Figure 27.11

   a. Describe the relationship between the uterine tubes and the uterus. How
      is this different from the relationship between the uterine tubes and the
      ovaries?

   b. Which image depicts a clearer interaction between the two?

5. **CD: Reproductive System > Female Flythrough (during oocyte development)**

   Textbook: Figure 27.12

   a. Describe the stages of the ovarian cycle, as seen in these images. How does ovulation occur?

   b. What are the advantages of each of these depictions of the ovarian cycle?

Multiple Choice

This section gives you an opportunity to demonstrate your understanding of the material covered in this workbook and in the text. Circle the correct answer for each question.

1. **The correct pathway of sperm through the male system from formation to ejaculation is**

   a. seminiferious tubule > ductus deferens > epididymis > ejaculatory duct.
   b. ductus deferens > ejaculatory duct > seminiferous tubule > epididymis.
   c. seminiferous tubule > ejaculatory duct > epididymis > ductus deferens.
   d. seminiferous tubule > epididymis > ductus deferens > ejaculatory duct.

2. **The gland(s) responsible for the production of a fructose-rich fluid comprising 60% of the total semen volume is/are the**

   a. seminal vesicles.
   b. prostate gland.
   c. endometrial glands.
   d. bulbourethral glands.

3. **Sperm undergo spermiogenesis and maturation in the**

   a. ductus deferens.
   b. epididymus.
   c. sustentacular cells.
   d. spermatogonia.

4. **The prostate gland produces**

   a. a weak acid.
   b. prostatic fluid.
   c. seminalplasmin.
   d. all of the above.

5. **Immediately before exiting the testes, sperm pass through the**
   a. seminiferous tubules.
   b. efferent ducts of the testes.
   c. rete testes.
   d. testicular lobules.

6. **The structure that holds the oocyte immediately prior to ovulation is the**

   a. Graafian follicle.
   b. primordial follicle.
   c. secondary follicle.
   d. corpus luteum.

7. **The superior portion of the uterus is referred to as the**

   a. os.
   b. cervix.
   c. fundus.
   d. body.

8. **The organ upon which the uterus rests is the**

   a. sigmoid colon.
   b. anus.
   c. ischium.
   d. urinary bladder.

9. **The correct sequence through which the oocyte passes upon ovulation is**

   a. fimbria > cervix > vagina > ampulla of uterine tube.
   b. fimbria > ampulla of uterine tube > cervix > vagina.
   c. ampulla of uterine tube > fimbria > cervix > vagina.
   d. ampulla of uterine tube > cervix > fimbria > vagina.

10. **The ovaries are held in place by the**

   a. broad ligament.
   b. round ligament.
   c. ovarian ligament.
   d. both B and C are correct.